# *You've Got a Friend*

## A Journal of Hope for Women with Breast Cancer

# You've Got a Friend

## A Journal of Hope for Women with Breast Cancer

*Yvonne Buchanan-Manley, RN, BS, MA*

HATHERLEIGH PRESS
NEW YORK

Hatherleigh Press
5–22 46th Avenue
Long Island City, NY 11101
1-800-528-2550
www.hatherleighpress.com

The patients represented in this book are composites of many people and ideas.
They do not represent specific individuals, either living or dead.

The ideas and suggestions contained in this book are not intended as a substitute for consulting with a physician. All matters regarding your health require medical supervision.

Library of Congress Cataloging-in-Publication Data
TO COME



Designed by Dede Cummings Designs
Printed in Canada on acid-free paper
10 9 8 7 6 5 4 3 2 1 ♾

*Weeping may endure for a night, but joy cometh in the morning.*

–Psalms 31:5

*To give…beauty for ashes, the oil of joy for mourning, the garment of praise for the spirit of heaviness…* –Isaiah 61:3

*Who is he that hideth counsel without knowledge? Therefore have I uttered that I understood not;*
*things too wonderful for me, which I knew not.* –Job 42:3

*So the Lord blessed the latter end of Job more than his beginning…* –Job 42:12

*My grace is sufficient for thee: for my strength is made perfect in weakness…*–Corinthians 12:9

# Dedication

This book is first dedicated to women with breast cancer, and to Adrienne Polon, health clinician, who cared for me expertly. My special thanks to: Robert Abrams, MD; David Becker, MD; Anthony Cahan, MD; Stanley Dauber, DPM; Helen DeRosis, MD; Stewart Fleishman, MD; Alan Freidman, MD; Robert Freidman, MD; Kenneth Greenspan, MD; Harry Gruenspan, MD, PhD; Joseph Iraci, MD; Robert Knapp, MD; Lynn Ratner, MD; Roy Schoen, MD; David Slavit, MD; Leonard Lustgarten, MD; Michael Schmerin, MD; Steven Hurowitz, RPh, BA, BS; Lenox Hill Hospital; Lenox Hill Radiology; East River Medical Imaging; family and friends; to the people at Hatherleigh Press, Ltd. And to Kevin Moran of Hatherleigh Press, Ltd., who had faith in my first book and guided its publication; and to all the others who should be listed....

But it is most especially for Alan Douglas Heymann, MD, FACS, committed healer/surgeon and extraordinary human being, who gave me the best new beginning of my life.

# Contents

# About the Author

This book is the product of a very personal experience with breast cancer, and the author brings to it not only this, but also substantial experience as a healer. From beginning as a surgical, pediatric, then psychiatric nurse, she was a faculty member of Rutgers University College of Nursing at a time when the college set a pattern in nursing education, and Dr. Hildegarde Peplau, the initiator of psychiatric nursing programs at Columbia and Rutgers, was her mentor. She has done individual and group counseling for the past fifteen years, along with working in the medical community doing research with doctors to enhance doctor-doctor and doctor-patient communications. Her work with breast cancer was born of her own experience, knowing that she was "just a woman" facing this disease. The result, this book, has been lauded by a chief of breast surgery, an internationally known gynecologic oncologic surgeon who co-discovered the CA125 blood test for ovarian cancer, and an internationally known psychiatrist author. Most importantly, she brings to her work a very great love for people.

Yvonne's undergraduate work (RN BS) was at Washington University in St. Louis under the chancellorship of Dr. Arthur Holly Compton, Nobel laureate for the Compton effect in X-ray. She was heavily influenced by his saying, "The scientists, and I am one of them, do believe in miracles, for we have seen miracles and know how they work." Her graduate work (MA degree and PhD studies) at New York University was in Culture and Communication with major emphasis on group psychology. Her advisor and mentor there was Dr. Neil Postman, author of several books related to education, futurology, group psychology, and media ecology.

The present story started on a bright July day in 1996, when Yvonne went for routine yearly mammogram and found that she had breast cancer. Subsequent lumpectomy, then mastectomy, followed. She is "counting down" five years on tamoxifen, with one year more to take it. This leads her to emphasize that our focus should be, not on the physical, which is different for each of us, but on the body/mind experience which has some surprisingly common elements, as well as individual elements. *Her basic philosophy is that one can focus on healing rather than fear.* She says, "We may have to have breast cancer, we may even have to die of breast cancer, but we can choose our reactions to it, and avoid the morbid approach so popular in the media."

Yvonne is from Missouri ("you have to show her"), she is twice widowed, her children are a couple of "adoptees" and her Godchild. She is active in a multitude of community activities and plays the flute. She can be found at synagogue on Friday evenings and church on Sundays, and has broad ecumenical interests.

*Above all, she brings you very great love, and after the weeping, joy!*

# Introduction

*"Courage is the resistance to fear, mastery of fear—not absence of fear."*
– Mark Twain

*"Hope is an adventure, a going forward—a confident search for a rewarding life."*
– Karl Menninger

These are two of many quotes which helped me during my own recent experience with cancer of the breast. They serve as an introduction to some feelings I offer you on the subject.

It is important to note that this is just my experience, which may or may not be the same as yours. Since we are all different, our experiences vary. However, in the hope that some common threads may be helpful, this book will tell you some thoughts that occurred to me.

It has been one of the most emotional experiences of my life. I have learned to honor and express those emotions. In the process, I have grown, and become an even more open person. If it is possible to turn adversity to advantage, I found this an opportunity to try to do so. The diagnosis was shocking and I could choose to stay in the almost surrealistic shock, or hell, that this brought to mind, or use it as a springboard for a new perspective and beginning. I, early on, chose the new beginning, and for me it has made all the difference. It should be said this is not a smooth ride to newness, but that it has ups and downs.

I heard all sorts of different statements about this disease from non-medical sources. This was frightening and confusing. The more "medical" writings on the subject were a bit more than I could concentrate on. I decided to respect my own feelings and decisions about my situation, deal only with direct professional advice, and to let others take their own path. You may wish to do it differently.

It would be my very great privilege to walk with you a little along this path we share together, and to hope that I have at least partially understood what you may be feeling.

It so happens that I am a nurse, but during this experience I was just a woman—and part of the very special sisterhood that you and I and others are in. And we will respect and feel for each other before we move along. And move along we must, for that is freedom, healing and life.

# *Part 1:*
# FEELINGS

*You are invited to write your thoughts, feelings, poems, and/or to draw on this page.*

Early in my breast cancer experience I made the remark that it was a roller coaster ride. It struck me that this was an appropriate expression of the feeling, from the beginning and through the recovery period, that you are fine, or better than usual, followed by a time of feeling tired, overwhelmed and exhausted. One woman said to me, "I just don't care," meaning that she was for that moment in time on overload since she went on to cite a number of things she did care about. This feeling may indicate a need to rest, take a deep breath, and allow yourself to feel tired. If it does not lift you may want to consider counseling.

Enjoy and savor those times, which also will come, when you feel the power of healing, nurturing and kindness. Because they are likely to be there in abundance. This can happen when someone does something for you, when you feel something in common with someone, when you just feel better for no discernible reason.

No, things will never be the same. But the different future may turn out to be richer than the past. Let yourself feel. Don't turn it off.

The roller coaster may continue for a long time. We are more vulnerable now, although in many ways stronger.

*You are invited to write your thoughts, feelings, poems, and/or to draw on this page.*

What are bridges? Things connecting one thing to another. Friends are the greatest bridges, but some of this path may need to be traveled alone. Some of us need more time alone than others.

For me, it was necessary to remove myself somewhat to be alone to think about what was happening and what I wanted to do. I have always been that type of person. Facing what was happening, *for me,* could best be done without any tranquilizers, antidepressants, or other things to take the edge off. It was painful sometimes, but always produced a resulting tranquility from which I felt that I could function through this.

Certainly, the help of medical personnel—ranging from physicians to the person who cleans in the hospital—can be enormously important to the continuity of care and well-being. For me, the surgeon and his office manager were enormously comforting. Other relationships varied according to the way I presented myself to the people around me.

There are people who are "born bridges," I found. They will come into your life expectedly or unexpectedly. Be very grateful for them. You will recognize them. It can change your life.

As time goes on, you will find more bridges, feel a fellowship with mankind you have not felt before, which is a transforming experience

*You are invited to write your thoughts, feelings, poems, and/or to draw on this page.*

One thing at a time, or one day at a time, have become common sayings in support groups. The value of taking one day at a time in dealing with breast cancer is that it feels overwhelming to do otherwise. Also, global thinking about it tends to immobilize us and stop us from reasoning things out and making the decisions we need to make for ourselves.

This is not just true for the time when you first hear that you have breast cancer, and have been told your options, but throughout the treatment, recovery and progress to the future.

Priorities enter into this. What things do you have to consider? What actions do you need to take? What kind of window of time is available in which you can make your decision—what are the time limits on your decision-making? The floor that does not get mopped will still be there when you get around to it.

One good gauge of priorities is to think of the decision that is bothering you most and try to deal with that first. Another school of thought says take care of small nagging concerns first, and then be free to focus on the larger ones. I found that, in this situation, I tended to do well in facing head-on and thinking of the things that bothered me most first.

You may want to make lists to help with this process. Sometimes a friend can see more clearly what needs to be done next, and next, and next. I was blessed to have a friend who led me through this priority of needs when I felt overwhelmed because she had been through it herself.

Know that the medical follow-up, as months and years go on, may become trying. A series of medical appointments and tests reaching far into the future may seem overwhelming. For me, waiting is devastating; so I plan to do constructive and positive thinking during these times of waiting. Know that the appointments are your medical link to continued health, and you can do it.

*You are invited to write your thoughts, feelings, poems, and/or to draw on this page.*

Why someone did not ask me to open my mouth so that they could see the motor, I don't know. I talked and talked and talked nonstop, with the feeling of needing to get all of this said. Part of this was a cover for what I was really feeling of good positive emotions which I was too shy to express.

In any case, there was a feeling of being "wound up," and that there was a necessity to "talk it out."

I noticed that some other women seemed to go silent. Whether they were too depressed to talk, or were quiet by nature, or just not ready to talk about their experience, I don't know. *But it is crucially important not to build a wall shutting out feelings. Talk it out.*

Generally, it seems that there may be a tendency to talk much more or less, than before we are faced with this experience. Probably, the talking more is a better safety valve, against the possibility of severe depression, for the churning emotions bound to be related to breast cancer. In either case, you are not alone in the experience of change in the amount of talking.

One woman I counseled hardly spoke at all. Finally she said, "My mind is so confused." I said, "Would the word terrified describe it better?" She said, "Yes, yes. I need to talk to you!" And we made great progress from this point about healing her fears.

*You are invited to write your thoughts, feelings, poems, and/or to draw on this page.*

Somewhere we have heard that we are "supposed" to be angry about this. It amazed me that I was not angry. I found that I actually was *very* angry. I was angry at the loss of a breast although I knew intellectually that it was the best choice for me.

This anger was expressed in saying some very critical things about almost everything, in a somewhat arrogant way. Also, in speaking to friends, and feeling anger at some of their remarks which would not have angered me before. Caution here—I also learned some of my friends' and relatives' worst qualities, which for some reason had not been clear before the change in me, but in turn felt more forgiving in weighing the positives and negatives. What about my own "worst" qualities? They came out in impatience, angry tears, depressed negative feelings, bitchiness—any number of vents for my emotions. A bravado and boastfulness covered my feelings of inadequacy and loss. This too will heal.

What were the positive qualities? Enhanced bravery, compassion, persistence, resiliency, resourcefulness. You will find these increased too, probably along with other qualities that belong to you alone. Probably, we will be blessed with more compassion too.

Recognizing what we are doing and how we are behaving with our anger can help us to express anger appropriately and to see its converse side, peace and joy.

*You are invited to write your thoughts, feelings, poems, and/or to draw on this page.*

People who have just had lumpectomy may feel damaged and hurt. Those of us who have experienced mastectomy have sustained a major loss not unlike bereavement, whether we have reconstruction or not.

A woman who runs a boutique for women with breast cancer in a major medical center in New York surprised me and set lights flashing in my head when I asked her if she had ever seen anyone satisfied with their reconstruction or prosthesis. Without hesitation she said she had not.

I had seen the sculpted-perfect four-stage reconstruction in a professional woman who had had mastectomy. Four stages to get it to her liking. She talked about the difference in sensation between the reconstructed breast and the remaining one, and was saddened that she could not feel the sensation in the reconstructed breast, with her husband, that she had felt before. Although another woman who had reconstruction said, "My boyfriend can't tell the difference." The unspoken rest of her hesitation there may be that *she* could tell the difference. Sensation may also return.

At present four years post-mastectomy, I have not yet had reconstruction and don't know whether or not I will. The sensation on my mastectomized side is a nipple-like sensation that I would not like to lose. This is a very individual decision, and you must be the one to decide. If you feel very ambivalent, or are very depressed about it, you may need to seek counseling.

But I believe, whether or not reconstruction is selected, we all mourn the loss of a breast. We may go through stages of denial (even feeling a "phantom" breast as if the breast were still there),

*You are invited to write your thoughts, feelings, poems, and/or to draw on this page.*

anger ("Why did this happen to me? Instead of why *not* me"), bargaining (as in a reconstruction of several stages to get back what was lost), and finally acceptance.

How do we mourn before we can accept? We face the fact, look our pain in the eye instead of avoiding it, admit it and try to be open about it, allow ourselves anger without criticizing ourselves for it, and understand that although we will never have the breast back we are still whole and likely to be better people for the experience. And again looking our pain in the eye, know that we can have reconstruction or a prosthesis, both of which, to the rest of the world, look miraculously natural even in a bathing suit. The breast may be gone, but love and enjoy the new you.

It helped me to touch my chest as soon as it was healed, get acquainted with it and let the warmth of my hand comfort.

*You are invited to write your thoughts, feelings, poems, and/or to draw on this page.*

The first concern for treating and getting rid of the cancer, and having it treated, later gives way to concern for survival and quality of life. Discussion with one's physician as to treatment, follow-up and prognosis will allay some of these fears. While being positive, there is a drive in me to look for certainty where certainty may not exist. This assumption changes to a new view of the fact that life has many uncertainties.

What to do? To look at friends, interests, and fun in a new way. To feel deserving of new experiences. To live one day at a time looking forward to the future with hope.

New interests and new friends may develop during this period, and certainly every day brings a new joy in being alive.

*You are invited to write your thoughts, feelings, poems, and/or to draw on this page.*

It is natural that there be some concern as to how men will react to the absence of a breast. It is a major sexual organ, as well as a symbol of feminine appearance and body symmetry.

There will of course be some difference in this concern according to the women's current relationships. I was widowed at the time this happened to me. I know that he would have accepted this with compassion, great empathy, and concern, feeling that my essence was still the same as before. For women who are in the dating process, there is concern as to how men will feel. Also, there is the question of when to tell them.

Among the men friends that I knew at the time I was about to have surgery, there was interest but platonic relationships. Even though these relationships did not involve sexuality, since they were more of the brother-sister variety, there were quick expressions from the men.

To one friend, I said, "I am going to be as much of a woman with one breast as some women could be with three." I was angry and needed to feel this positively. Without missing a beat, he said, "Not as-much-of, more." Another friend kissed me on the cheek, not the least repulsed, and expressed his concern that I had not asked more help of him during my time in the hospital. Another prayed with me, held my hand, and was compassionate and upbeat. At some level, before these encounters, I had thought of lumpectomy or mastectomy as a turn-off for men in general.

We still wonder, how that would be, how we would feel, and how the man would feel. Also, there is a negative feeling—that we don't want to burden a new man with this disease and its uncertainty. On the other hand, life is uncertain, and this may not be a reason to let a man go.

Married women I have spoken with after their mastectomy tell me consistently that their

*You are invited to write your thoughts, feelings, poems, and/or to draw on this page.*

husbands were more attentive and compassionate after the surgery than before. One woman qualified this by saying, "Of course, he can walk away from it, and I can't." I felt that was being a little rough on the man, although I could understand what she might have been feeling. Know that the man suffers too, but his love for you doesn't depend on whether you have a breast(s) or not.

When to tell a new man? I would guess that some balance needs to be struck here, where we each figure out what is best for us individually. Some people feel that you should wait for the relationship to get "serious" before telling a man about the mastectomy. On the other hand, there may be some advantages to an earlier brief mention, to clear the air for both yourself and the man so that the relationship can progress, or gently end if the man can't accept the idea of mastectomy. Overall, I have been reassured that compassion and acceptance seem to prevail, and know that the woman's ability to love and feel sexually attracted may indeed increase rather than decrease after mastectomy.

*You are invited to write your thoughts, feelings, poems, and/or to draw on this page.*

This probably differs considerably from individual to individual. For me the major "can't talk about it" was the idea that maybe both breasts should be taken off at the same time, since I had been told that both breasts had a lumpy consistency, although only one contained the cancer. Even though I knew that I could not have done this either emotionally or physically, it still haunted me. Then I realized that if this was a valid option, my surgeon would have discussed it with me—so here and throughout, *I learned that trust in your physician is something you must decide on and go with.* Also, don't be afraid to say what you are thinking. You may think it silly or stupid, but it is not, as long as it concerns you. Remember that your surgeon is not clairvoyant. He also can be trusted to tell you if your thinking is going out in left field.

One woman I spoke with said that she was unable to think about the possibility that having several women in her family with breast cancer meant that she might have it.

One helpful exercise may be to write down those things that you are not able to say. This gets the thoughts from head to paper and may give you a different perspective. *Also, not being able to talk about it now does not mean you can't talk about it later.*

The major "can't-talk-about-it" is probably the possibility of death. It might be better not to isolate breast cancer as a reason for death, because we know that we are part of a stream of life in which everyone dies. Currently available media information can be inaccurate, morbid and depressing; it seems we only hear the sad stories, even though 20 plus years of survival are not uncommon now. We must do the best we can and live each minute to the fullest, surrounding ourselves with hope.

*You are invited to write your thoughts, feelings, poems, and/or to draw on this page.*

There may be an initial tendency not to tell anyone other than those closest to you about this experience, and even to limit that number. This was true for me at first because although I am a very gregarious person, I am also very private.

Once you decide to talk with people about it, you may be surprised at the positive response. As a rule of thumb, tell those people you want to tell, and intuitively know those you may not want to tell—such as employers in a very rigid work situation. You may even find that you want to remove yourself from that rigid situation.

While people will generally be sympathetic, as with any other disease, you will want to be careful about your timing. Since this has been such an enormous experience in your life, there may be a tendency to be too prolonged and detailed in your discussion. You know the old saying, that no one wants to hear the details of an operation, especially in a social setting.

You might also feel, as I did, a bit of impatience with people who complain about minor illnesses. I tried to be especially sympathetic, knowing that to some people a minor illness may be a major issue for reasons unknown to me. As a rule of thumb, brevity is the soul of wit and frequently of wisdom when it comes to telling people about your operation. Don't tell people whom you know to be morbid and negative. Do share with positive thinkers.

*You are invited to write your thoughts, feelings, poems, and/or to draw on this page.*

Along the way, we may doubt the validity of our thoughts about the situation. It is a lot to assimilate. Am I right about this? Am I wrong about that? And other feelings of uncertainty may come to mind.

We may even doubt the validity of our feelings. So much media experience may have given us the idea that there is something we are "supposed" to feel or "expected" to feel—or worse, that there is some encyclopedic book to memorize in order to do it right. The more that idea can be replaced by letting yourself think and feel naturally may make things a little easier to deal with. "Doing it right" is *your* way of feeling comfortable in dealing with a situation.

Also, it is possible that uncertainty is a result of "overload." It may be helpful to sit back, listen to music, take a walk, or anything else that seems helpful in freeing yourself of persistent uncertainty for a while, so that you can come back to your decision-making refreshed and more confident. Remember to take one thing at a time.

Expressing our thoughts to someone, particularly someone now recovered from similar experience, may be helpful, especially if you have a positive, stable friend who has walked this path earlier. If any group or individual is the right one to talk with, you will know it, because you will feel comfortable and right in the discussion—and nurtured. A word of caution: I attended one group meeting where I got the very uncomfortable feeling that the group was not only unhelpful, but was harmful *for me*. This was compounded by the fact that inaccurate medical information was dispensed, and the meetings were led by people who were not professionals. The bottom line is that being around anyone who takes a morbid attitude about breast cancer, or who isolates breast

*You are invited to write your thoughts, feelings, poems, and/or to draw on this page.*

cancer patients from the rest of the stream of life, or who has an attitude of resignation, is not helpful, and may be depressing at best. We are not waiting for the other shoe to fall; we are busy living to the fullest.

You may want to have at least one session with a psychiatrist about this. The complexity of the situation is enough to deal with without exposing yourself to negatives—don't be afraid to disagree and walk away if you feel a discussion is harmful to you. Also, don't be afraid to change your mind.

Above all, be doubtful of individuals or groups offering non-traditional miracle cures. I attended one large meeting in which the group was told that the doctor's vitamins were the way to go, rather than surgery, chemotherapy or radiation. A lovely woman I was counseling at the time was quite confused and hurt by this, and it negatively affected her recovery.

*You are invited to write your thoughts, feelings, poems, and/or to draw on this page.*

We may feel a great deal more vulnerable than usual for quite a while both before and after surgery. The sense of shock and loss may vary from one person to another, but certainly there is a feeling of hypersensitivity to one's surroundings.

You may feel more tearful than usual, and start feeling emotional during conversations with people when these feelings would not have produced the same reaction before. Your feelings may be more easily hurt than before. You may not feel as attractive as usual when you don't feel well. These feelings will pass, and hopefully will be replaced by even stronger positive feelings than before.

Be very good to yourself when you are feeling vulnerable in any way. Do things that comfort you. You may want to wear a favorite gown, robe, or other clothing to boost the spirits—very feminine underwear was a particular boost to me. Or listening to music, reading material appealing to you, playing a musical instrument (if you played one before), or dancing slowly to pleasant music may work, too. Generally, anything that gives you pleasure. One word of warning! Excess food or alcohol intake is not an appropriate way of getting pleasure.

I used these feelings of vulnerability to allow myself to speak more freely to people around me. It also may help to forewarn friends that you might be a little more cross, edgy, or tearful than usual for a while, and to ask them to bear with you. Sometimes there is a feeling of diminished control over events which may also affect this feeling, so try to focus on those things that you can control. There are always options. Even though they may not be numerous, they are there—and probably more available than you may think.

*You are invited to write your thoughts, feelings, poems, and/or to draw on this page.*

There is a very great need to feel loved and protected during this difficult time of your life. But the other side of the coin is that you will probably find more loving support and compassion surrounding you than you ever dreamed possible, along with an enormous sense of gratitude.

You may not notice this caring until all of a sudden you are aware of the unusual number of people who have shown you caring, kindness, compassion and love. These things came to me from new people in my life, from close friends, and from people I had not seen or heard from in a long, long time.

Do not forget self-love in this process. It is okay to give yourself credit for coming through a most trying situation with at least some flying colors. Appreciate that and applaud yourself for it. Surprisingly, self-esteem and the ability to love might even increase as time goes on.

*You are invited to write your thoughts, feelings, poems, and/or to draw on this page.*

One of the most surprising aspects of this experience, to me, was feeling more feminine afterward than
I had before. The hows and whys are difficult to describe, but you may have a similar experience.

*Most of the women I know who have had breast cancer tell stories about some kind of a lack of nurturing earlier.* Perhaps they had a history of breaking up with a man they loved very much or a husband who was not very attentive. They may have devoted considerable effort to being the strong one in a situation in which numerous children, their husband, or other relatives needed or demanded an inordinate amount of attention.

Now is the time to recognize and sort out any feelings of this sort, and focus on your personal growth and a new perspective about loving. You may find this happening spontaneously or you may want to seek counseling. Perhaps this question does not apply to your situation. By all means, learn to nurture yourself in every possible way, because it is healing and may open new doors for you. How to nurture? Be good to yourself, reduce demands on yourself unless they are positive and lead to growth, and do things that give you pleasure.

*You are invited to write your thoughts, feelings, poems, and/or to draw on this page.*

This is a somewhat fearful time and one major source of the sense of being loved and protected is from the faith you may have in God. Yes, don't be afraid to say it.

For myself, this was not a new part of my life because I had been born into a religious home, and following a college-age period of agnosticism had become firmly ecumenical. Just before I was taken into surgery, I told the doctors and nurses around me that we were covered with a big prayer blanket, that I was an Episcopalian, and that in addition, Roman Catholic, Jewish, various Protestant, and Buddhist prayers were being said for us. Last but not least, I told them, we were being prayed for by a man who had graduated from MIT and had a doctorate in theology—I thought he might know the "best route."

An Episcopal priest from my parish visited me in the hospital and talked with me several times both before and after surgery. If you don't have a religious affiliation, the hospital will always have a chaplain whom you can ask for if you wish, and New York City is probably unique in having the HealthCare Chaplaincy which teaches chaplains and represents more than thirty different faiths.

Frequent attendance at church and synagogue has become my habit. One gift from synagogue is the prayer, *"When we despair, open our hearts to joy."*

*You are invited to write your thoughts, feelings, poems, and/or to draw on this page.*

As said before, you may want at least one session with a psychiatrist or allied kind of counselor early on. Also, if you find your "roller coaster" going on longer than you wish or if you feel prolonged severe depression, you will want help with this. It can be not only healing, but also a boost to your spirits.

You may ask your internist or your surgeon for a referral, or you may find a counselor through a recognized clinic or through the local mental health association.

It is in no way a "failure" to seek this kind of assistance if you feel that you need it.

There are also support groups you may want to consider that are attended by women who have been through similar experiences. Choose these carefully, for a positive approach rather than random catharsis and playing "Ain't it awful?" My organization, Renaissance: A New Beginning, offers counseling.

We need positive nurturing now. It has been my observation that part of our sisterhood is that we have experienced negative nurturing before our cancer—from family, spouse, lover or any significant other.

*You are invited to write your thoughts, feelings, poems, and/or to draw on this page.*

This may be a time when you will want, at some point, to review from a new perspective the personal characteristics that are part of you. In a sense, you may want to clean and clear your emotional "closet," softening some unwanted traits and enhancing more positive ones.

For me, it was a surprise to find myself acting highly critical and judgmental, and a further surprise to find that this was not an entirely new part of me. I learned that I too had made mistakes and that others have a right to their opinions, and may have totally different views than myself with complete validity.

On the other hand, I found that I had often accepted more criticism of myself than was justified, and I was surprised to find how some people I had known a long time made attempts to direct and control me.

From all of this grew a new tolerance and a parallel self-protectiveness. There is no time like the present, and the breast cancer experience certainly may teach us that now is the time to be ourselves since each moment has become more precious.

*You are invited to write your thoughts, feelings, poems, and/or to draw on this page.*

You may not sleep well even after you've made your bedroom a happy, peaceful and colorful place. We all know that problems seem worse in the middle of the night than at any other time. Be patient with yourself. You have been through hell and you will come through to the light.

What might you think about at 4 am? Money? Pain? Relationships? Your lost or damaged breast, and the nightmarish quality of the loss? The people in your life? Your safety? Whether or not you will live? Whether the man in your life will be sad, frightened, or turned off? What about your work? And on and on it goes.

Know that we all share this experience with each other, and know that we are all loved. Above all, look your demons in the eye. They are not so terrifying then, and it may surprise you that healthy solutions occur to you. *We can't successfully run from terror, but we can walk through it to the other side.*

You also may want to re-focus. For example, instead of "What about my work?" think about what work you would like to do, which may be something different than what you have done. Think of something you have enjoyed in the past, or hope to enjoy in the future.

You might want to have a small earphone radio or tape player with you in bed, to hear news, commentary or music. Or you may want to play a tape of soothing sounds such as ocean waves, rain or porpoise sounds. Maybe you will like turning on the light, walking around, and getting a soda or a glass of milk.

Be good to yourself. Know that the light will come with dawn; that the dawn means new beginnings, and that just as surely as the dawn comes each day, there will be a new dimension to go

*You are invited to write your thoughts, feelings, poems, and/or to draw on this page.*

on to after this life. *Weeping may last for the night, but joy comes in the morning, as the Psalmist says.*

*Love yourself and others. Refuse to be morbid! We may have to have breast cancer, we may even die of breast cancer, but we can choose not to be morbid about it.*

*You are invited to write your thoughts, feelings, poems, and/or to draw on this page.*

Having always been in a medically related profession, I found my interest in and abilities in this area greatly enhanced. My professional life became much more gratifying. There is enormous satisfaction in feeling that we have helped someone else.

Others have expressed the wish to help others, especially other women with similar experiences. This may be done on a friend-to-friend basis, or through support groups for women who have had this experience. The more we stick to feelings rather than details and comparisons of physical experience, the more we will be helpful. Renaissance: A New Beginning is a support system I developed as a professional counselor who also had breast cancer. It can be reached by writing the author in care of Hatherleigh Press at Suite 200, 5–22 46th Avenue, Long Island City, NY 11101. Please enclose a self-addressed stamped envelope.

*You are invited to write your thoughts, feelings, poems, and/or to draw on this page.*

# *Part 2:*

# EVERYDAY THINGS

*You are invited to write your thoughts, feelings, poems, and/or to draw on this page.*

The old instruction from your relatives or teachers in childhood to stand up straight applies here. Having always had a tendency to slump somewhat, I found myself doing it more in compensation for the absence of one breast. Standing straight is important to our recovery of balance, mood, and to the recovery of the muscles near the area of surgery.

Instead of compensating by slumping before the prosthesis or reconstruction is fitted, try layering your clothes. A jacket over a top. A sweater that is a bit baggy. A friend from Paris brought me a luxurious huge silk scarf, which I wore home from the hospital. It not only looked beautiful; it completely compensated for any imbalance of symmetry at that time.

*You are invited to write your thoughts, feelings, poems, and/or to draw on this page.*

Having read that one should take some bras to the fitting of the prosthesis, I took those I customarily wore—one brightly flowered, one light purple, and one navy. The fitter said these were "sexy," with a rather critical tone. Yes, they were and that is what I still like in a bra.

The first bra I was shown looked suitable for a member of the Green Bay Packers—not for me! Maybe some people would love it and feel that it was sporty. Another fitter asked if I wanted an orthopedic bra. I replied that I did not, and would not have one. Certainly if this became necessary for some reason, okay, but not as something to wear simply because I had a mastectomy.

There is no reason that you can't wear a bra that is feminine, sexy, comfortable, and colorful. Pick and choose. Maybe it can't be a bikini bra, but anything else is cool.

*You are invited to write your thoughts, feelings, poems, and/or to draw on this page.*

You may have a choice between being fitted with a breast form or having surgical reconstruction after mastectomy.

The reconstruction can be done at the time of mastectomy or for most of us at least, there is a window of time to have reconstruction later. This should be discussed early on with your surgeon.

If you opt for a breast form, as I did, you will need to seek a place for a fitting. For a smaller-breasted woman the fitting is easier, while for larger-breasted women like myself it may seem to require a knowledge of quantum physics. Do not despair if you experience my predicament—it can be resolved. I went to talk with four to six fitting places before I chose the one that finally fitted me for the form. Another word for the form is prosthesis, which is a word I dislike as too medical or orthopedic—I even preferred my own term for the form, *faux breast.* It helped me to focus on the feminine rather than the medical in this context.

What I expected to be an easy process was in fact more involved than expected. For me, the entire experience was traumatic until one fitter said, *"I'm not fitting you to the form; I'm fitting the form to you."* This was exactly what I needed to hear, for it had been my feeling with the others that I was being molded into a form, a new kind of bra, and a new way of handling my bras, rather than ascertaining what I felt my needs to be instead of what the fitter told me my needs were. The focus should be on *you* rather than the *form.* Of course, there is a union of these two things, but

*You are invited to write your thoughts, feelings, poems, and/or to draw on this page.*

part of the need for us to have a maximum of choices is filled by the caring kind of statement that was made to me.

What were my needs? To look as feminine as possible. To have a form as identical to my real breast as possible in size, flexibility and texture. To have the form fit into a reasonable array of feminine, sexy bras, even though I realized that because of my large breast size this probably would not be a "bikini" bra. Nice lacy, pastel and navy regular bras that fit the form were not difficult to find in major department stores. I even found a leopard-printed bra! It is a good idea to take a couple of these new bras along with you to the fitter, with the option of exchanging them if you are not keen on the fit of the particular bra to the form. The fitter can sew a pocket into the bra to fit the prothesis.

It seemed to me that it was a boost to have new bras. Some old bras were thrown away (it was probably time to toss them anyway). Some favorite ones were kept to adapt to use with the form. Generally, for me, I felt a need for newness to go with the new situation. It was part of my acceptance of change. Don't be reluctant to experiment with the new form and bras in much the same way as you try on clothes, with a smoothing there and a tuck here, until you achieve the fit you want of bra-to-form-to-you.

*You are invited to write your thoughts, feelings, poems, and/or to draw on this page.*

One of the things I wanted very much to do was to swim again. What would I do about the breast form? Would the bathing suit fit?

A suit with bra cups sewn in (not as common as formerly) is ideal for the woman with mastectomy. A cup can also be sewn into the suit. The form used in regular clothes can be used and carefully washed and rinsed afterward.

But what a bit of serendipity I accidentally discovered having been given a frilly ball-shaped plastic bath sponge at a party grab-bag exchange. This sponge, placed in the cup of the bathing suit, molds to the shape of the cup in the suit, and lacks the weight of the regular form.

The sponge can be molded to the shape of the other cup, or cut if you wish it to be smaller, to make for symmetry. And blessing of blessings, it does not absorb water like a regular sponge, so water is not pouring from it when you come out of the water.

For aesthetics sake, the bathing suit and sponge are washed in a bit of liquid soap and hung on the shower rod to dry. No laborious cleaning of your form and feeling uneasy as to whether it might come out of the suit, or be discolored by salt or chlorine.

This bit of serendipity gave me a tremendous boost, smile and smug sense of satisfaction.

Last but not least, the exercises given for your arms following mastectomy can be done very effectively in the pool without the pull of gravity, which makes a great difference in the ease of doing the exercise and increasing the range of motion.

*You are invited to write your thoughts, feelings, poems, and/or to draw on this page.*

A friend who had a mastectomy followed by chemotherapy and radiation for a very aggressive cancer more than ten years ago, now runs to England and California in her teaching chores as a chemist. Her husband is also a chemist, so one tends to have faith in the two of them when it comes to chemistry. (A word of caution: *don't* use any treatment without an okay from your surgeon.) This couple put me wise to the aloe plant. My first one was brought to me in the hospital so that I could get used to looking at it, make friends with it, and enjoy it in its pert yellow, green and white pot and check on possible future uses for it.

After the staples were removed and healing progressed, I was allowed by my surgeon to use aloe on the incision line and surrounding skin. How to do it?

The aloe plant, as you may know, has long leaves that are similar to other cactus plants. Cut a leaf off the plant near the base of the leaf with a sharp scissors. Then rinse it thoroughly under cold water and dry it with a paper towel. Then, on another paper towel, use a scissors to cut off the longitudinal edge of the leaf on both sides. After that, dissect the leaf in half along its width, cutting until you have separated the two halves of the leaf, leaving two flat surfaces sticky and watery with the clear aloe juices. Apply this directly to the skin of the incision line and the skin around it. There should not be any stinging sensation or other discomfort; as a matter of fact, a soothing sensation is produced, and the healing process may well be speeded by this substance.

Another word of caution. Many products for sale in stores have labels saying "100% Aloe Gel." On closer examination, the contents part of the label may list as many as six other ingredients. The plant is preferable for this reason.

*You are invited to write your thoughts, feelings, poems, and/or to draw on this page.*

Early on, I gathered a dozen pillows of various sizes, washed them in the washing machine, and plopped them on the bed. These can be bright colors or covered with the pillow slips you like.

Not only does this give a luxurious feeling of comfort and add color as well as femininity; it also has practical application. When you are first home from the hospital and want to rest your arm on pillows, there they are. When you want to lie on your side, pillows can go between the arms for more comfortable positioning.

As time goes on, they are a comfort in a situation in which your balance without the form may feel quite different from your "old self." Certainly, if you choose to have reconstruction, these may be an added comfort in the recovery process.

*You are invited to write your thoughts, feelings, poems, and/or to draw on this page.*

As part of the newness of your life, you may have mixed feelings about the old and the new in your home. For me, establishing order and gradually getting rid of clutter and old things I had been hanging onto was important and a source of comfort.

The idea of new arrangements or simplifying your surroundings may be appealing as well.

Even the location of bras and forms can be a source of change. Make a new beginning in your home as well as yourself.

*You are invited to write your thoughts, feelings, poems, and/or to draw on this page.*

Before this experience, I told people that I was congenitally allergic to exercise. A lot of excess weight resulted, so there was another reason for exercise.

The exercises for the breast area provided by the hospital or your doctor will be used according to whatever instructions given to you by your doctor. It is important that you wait for the surgeon's okay before beginning to exercise, and that you follow the exercise schedule you are given.

A pool, after healing is complete, may be a wonderful way to exercise the entire body, and particularly the back, which can become very tired.

Along with exercise, eating a variety of foods is desirable including fruits and vegetables. It is advisable to make your selections low in fat, and to avoid frequent use of smoked foods. Since I wanted to lose some extra weight, I reduced quantity of food and gave up sweets. As a result, I went from 187 pounds to 125 in a year's time. I used exercises given to me by a physical therapist, and later a book titled *Strong Women Stay Young* by Miriam E. Nelson PhD and Sarah Wernick, PhD recommended to me by a Harvard colleague.

You may want to ask your doctor to refer you to a nutritionist and/or physical therapist for help with exercise and fitness.

*You are invited to write your thoughts, feelings, poems, and/or to draw on this page.*

My life has been filled with music, and I still play the flute. If you play a musical instrument, how about doing it again now? Do you like dancing? Do it again.

Radio, CD, tape—whatever suits you—can be another soothing influence. I found Chopin sonatas, Beethoven symphonies, Telemann, and flute music with harp were great. Pick and choose what suits you. It is a time for choosing and for letting what you desire come true.

Go to the symphony, to concerts, to church or synagogue, or musical events. I found the singing of a Cantor tranquilizing, but a church choir somewhat funereal.

# *Part 3:*
# HEALING AND LAUGHTER

*You are invited to write your thoughts, feelings, poems, and/or to draw on this page.*

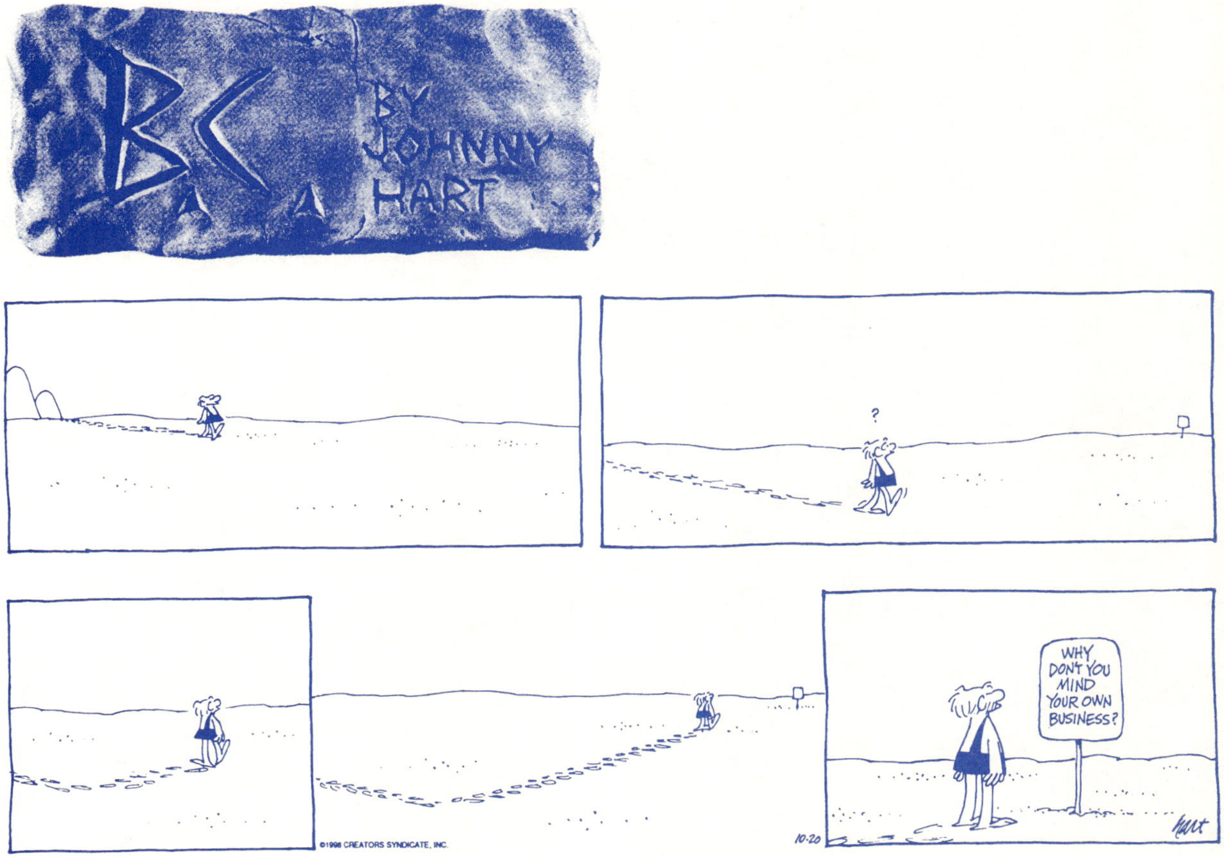
B.C.
BY JOHNNY HART
?
WHY DON'T YOU MIND YOUR OWN BUSINESS?
©1998 CREATORS SYNDICATE, INC.
10-20
hart

By permission of Johnny Hart and Creators Syndicate, Inc.

*You are invited to write your thoughts, feelings, poems, and/or to draw on this page.*

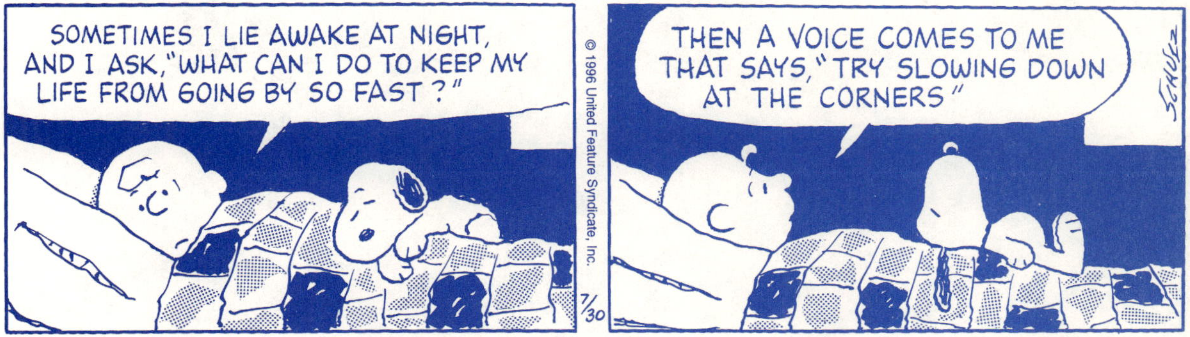
SOMETIMES I LIE AWAKE AT NIGHT, AND I ASK, "WHAT CAN I DO TO KEEP MY LIFE FROM GOING BY SO FAST ?"
© 1996 United Feature Syndicate, Inc.
7/30
THEN A VOICE COMES TO ME THAT SAYS, "TRY SLOWING DOWN AT THE CORNERS"
SCHULZ

PEANUTS reprinted by permission of United Features Syndicate, Inc.

*You are invited to write your thoughts, feelings, poems, and/or to draw on this page.*

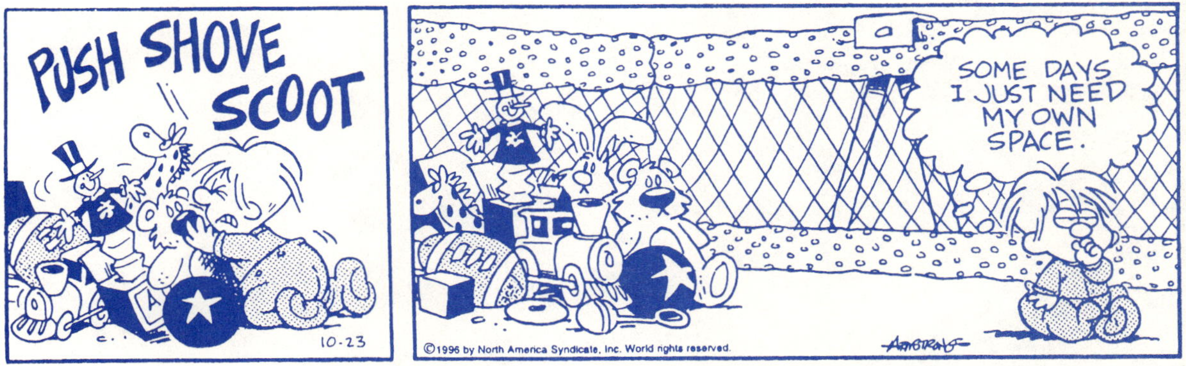


Reprinted with special permission of North American Syndicate.

*You are invited to write your thoughts, feelings, poems, and/or to draw on this page.*

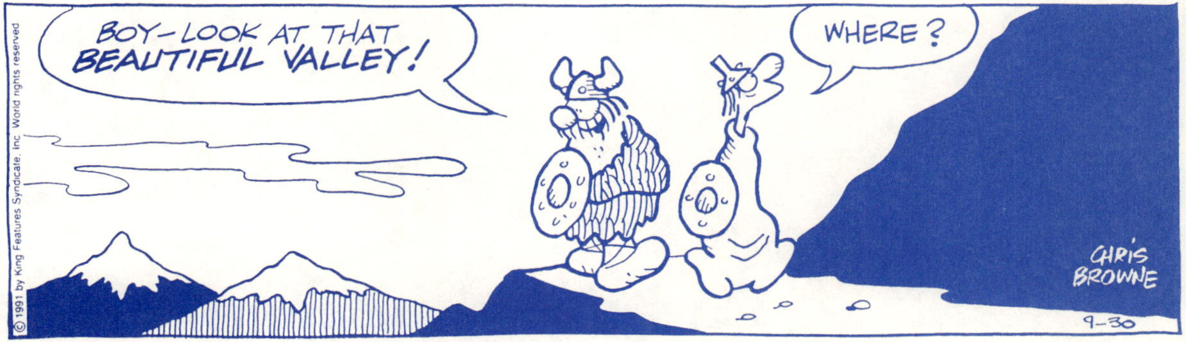
BOY-LOOK AT THAT BEAUTIFUL VALLEY!
WHERE?
CHRIS BROWNE
9-30
© 1991 by King Features Syndicate, Inc. World rights reserved

Reprinted with special permission of King Features Syndicate.

*You are invited to write your thoughts, feelings, poems, and/or to draw on this page.*

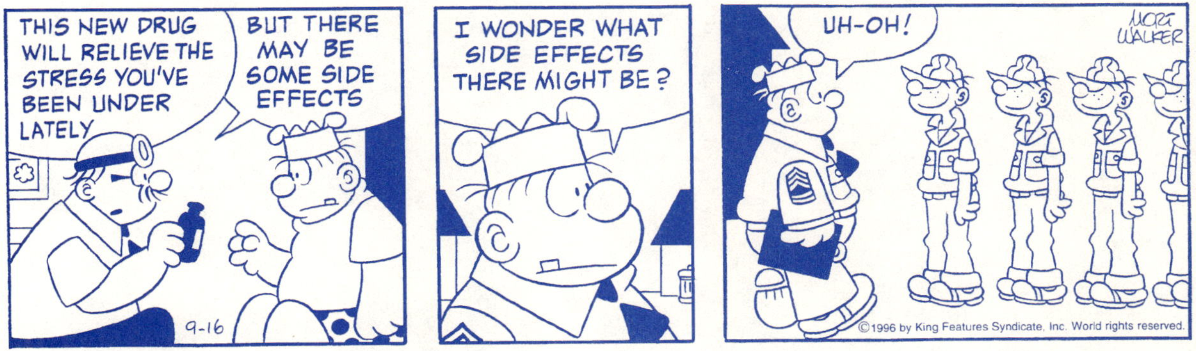
THIS NEW DRUG WILL RELIEVE THE STRESS YOU'VE BEEN UNDER LATELY
BUT THERE MAY BE SOME SIDE EFFECTS
9-16
I WONDER WHAT SIDE EFFECTS THERE MIGHT BE ?
UH-OH!
MORT WALKER
©1996 by King Features Syndicate, Inc. World rights reserved.

Reprinted with special permission of King Features Syndicate.

*You are invited to write your thoughts, feelings, poems, and/or to draw on this page.*

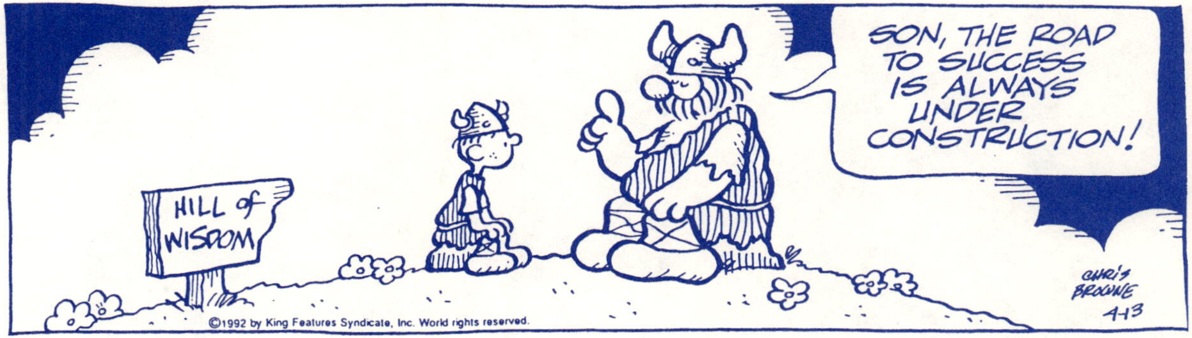
HILL of WISDOM
SON, THE ROAD TO SUCCESS IS ALWAYS UNDER CONSTRUCTION!
©1992 by King Features Syndicate, Inc. World rights reserved.
CHRIS BROWNE 4-13

Reprinted with special permission of King Features Syndicate.

*You are invited to write your thoughts, feelings, poems, and/or to draw on this page.*

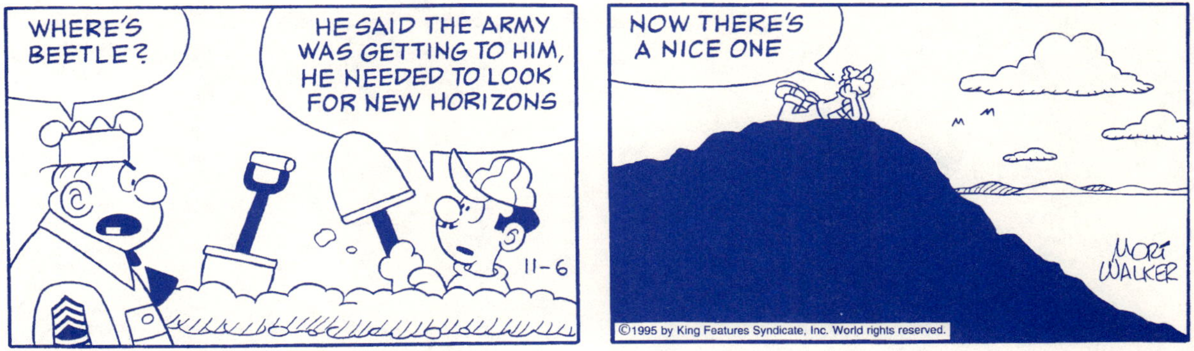
WHERE'S BEETLE?
HE SAID THE ARMY WAS GETTING TO HIM, HE NEEDED TO LOOK FOR NEW HORIZONS
11-6
NOW THERE'S A NICE ONE
MORT WALKER
©1995 by King Features Syndicate, Inc. World rights reserved.

Reprinted with special permission of King Features Syndicate.

*You are invited to write your thoughts, feelings, poems, and/or to draw on this page.*

**THE FAMILY CIRCUS®** **By Bil Keane**

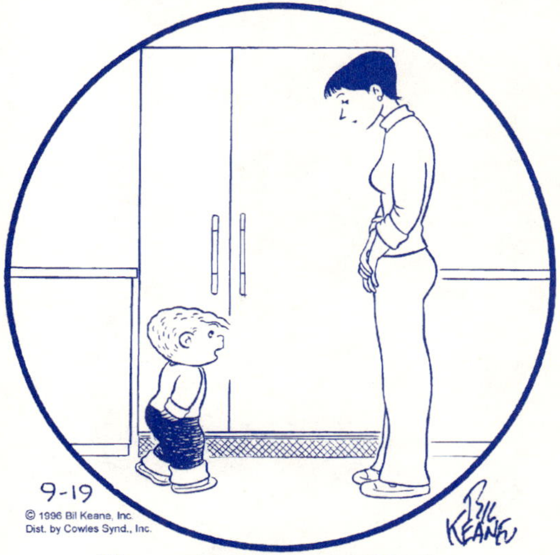


"I'm not hungry, or thirsty, or any of that stuff. What I'd REALLY like is a hug."

Reprinted with special permission of King Features Syndicate.

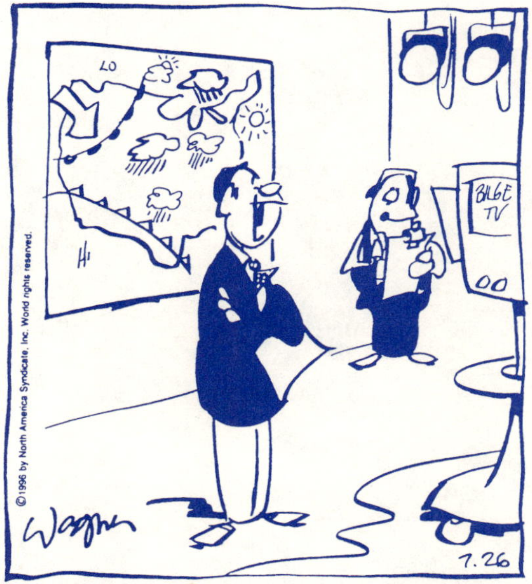


**"The weather advisory is: Direct your feet to the sunny side of the street."**

Reprinted with special permission of North American Syndicate.

*You are invited to write your thoughts, feelings, poems, and/or to draw on this page.*

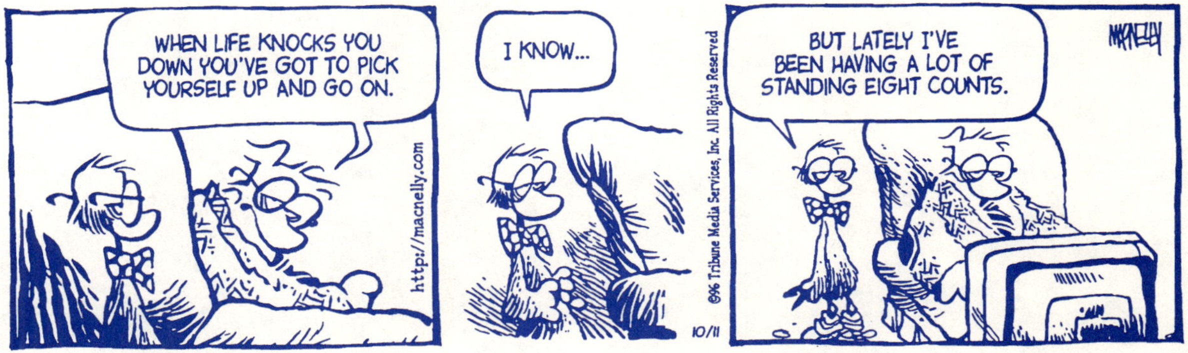
WHEN LIFE KNOCKS YOU DOWN YOU'VE GOT TO PICK YOURSELF UP AND GO ON.
http://macnelly.com
I KNOW...
©96 Tribune Media Services, Inc. All Rights Reserved
10/11
BUT LATELY I'VE BEEN HAVING A LOT OF STANDING EIGHT COUNTS.
MACNELLY

*You are invited to write your thoughts, feelings, poems, and/or to draw on this page.*

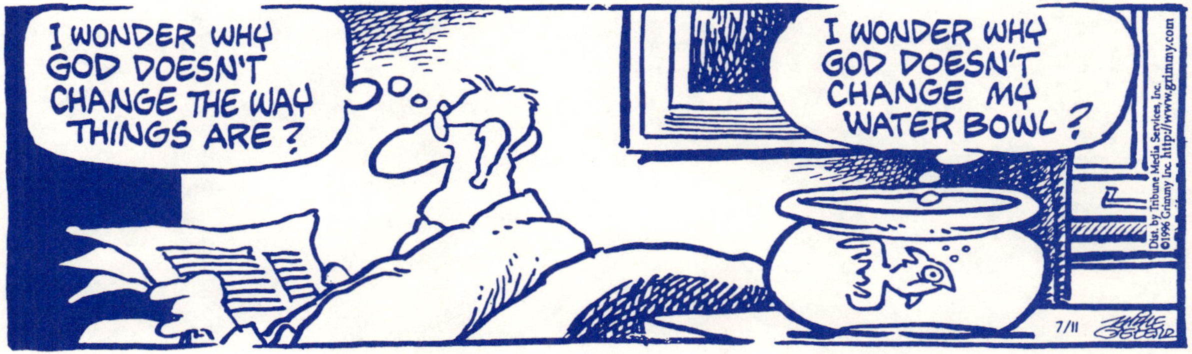
I WONDER WHY GOD DOESN'T CHANGE THE WAY THINGS ARE?
I WONDER WHY GOD DOESN'T CHANGE MY WATER BOWL?
Dist. by Tribune Media Services, Inc.
©1996 Grimmy Inc. http://www.grimmy.com
7/11

*You are invited to write your thoughts, feelings, poems, and/or to draw on this page.*

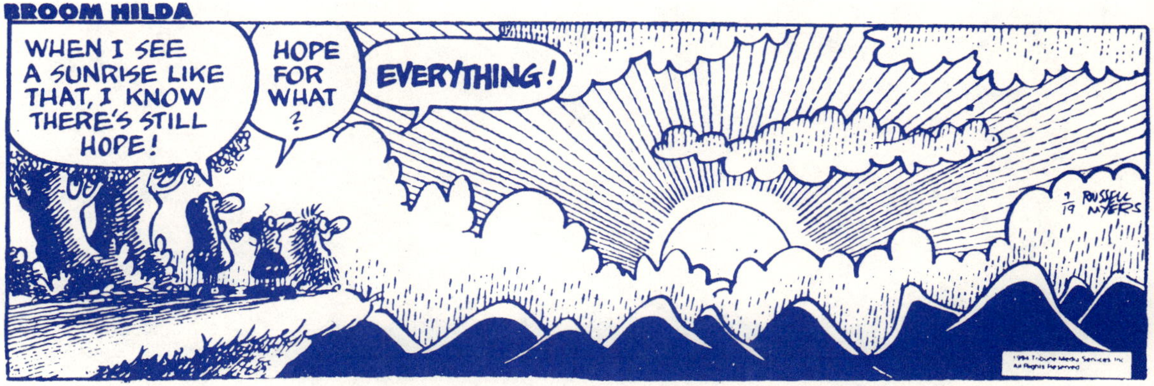
BROOM HILDA
WHEN I SEE A SUNRISE LIKE THAT, I KNOW THERE'S STILL HOPE!
HOPE FOR WHAT ?
EVERYTHING!
9 19 RUSSELL MYERS

*You are invited to write your thoughts, feelings, poems, and/or to draw on this page.*

**For Better or For Worse®** **by Lynn Johnston**

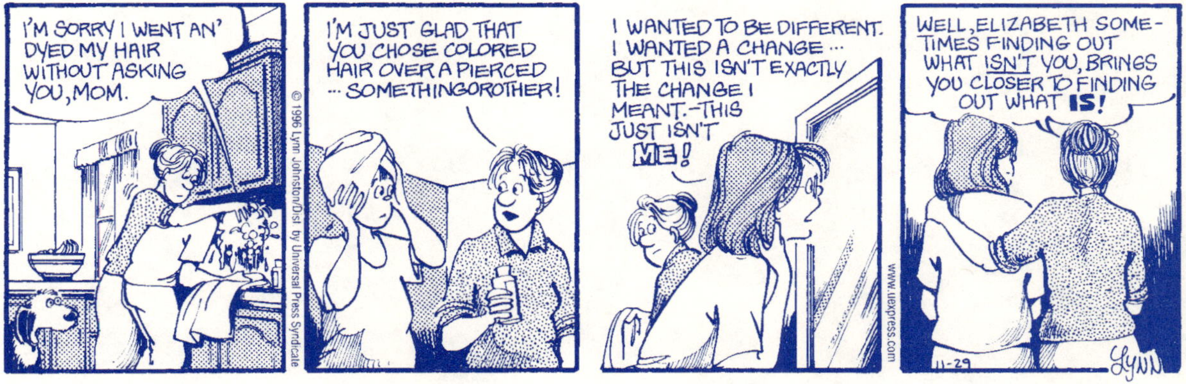

*You are invited to write your thoughts, feelings, poems, and/or to draw on this page.*

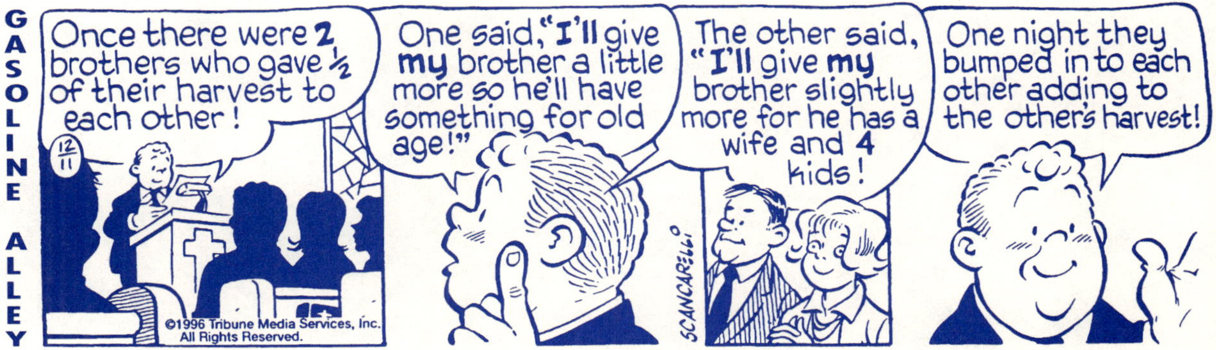
GASOLINE ALLEY
Once there were 2 brothers who gave ½ of their harvest to each other!
12/11
©1996 Tribune Media Services, Inc. All Rights Reserved.
One said, "I'll give my brother a little more so he'll have something for old age!"
The other said, "I'll give my brother slightly more for he has a wife and 4 kids!
SCANCARELLI
One night they bumped in to each other adding to the other's harvest!

*You are invited to write your thoughts, feelings, poems, and/or to draw on this page.*

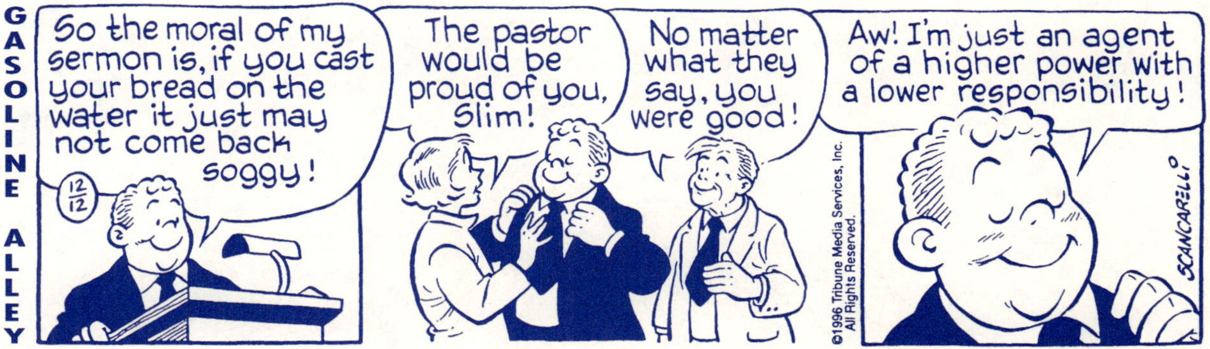
GASOLINE ALLEY
So the moral of my sermon is, if you cast your bread on the water it just may not come back soggy!
12/12
The pastor would be proud of you, Slim!
No matter what they say, you were good!
©1996 Tribune Media Services, Inc. All Rights Reserved.
Aw! I'm just an agent of a higher power with a lower responsibility!
SCANCARELLI

*You are invited to write your thoughts, feelings, poems, and/or to draw on this page.*

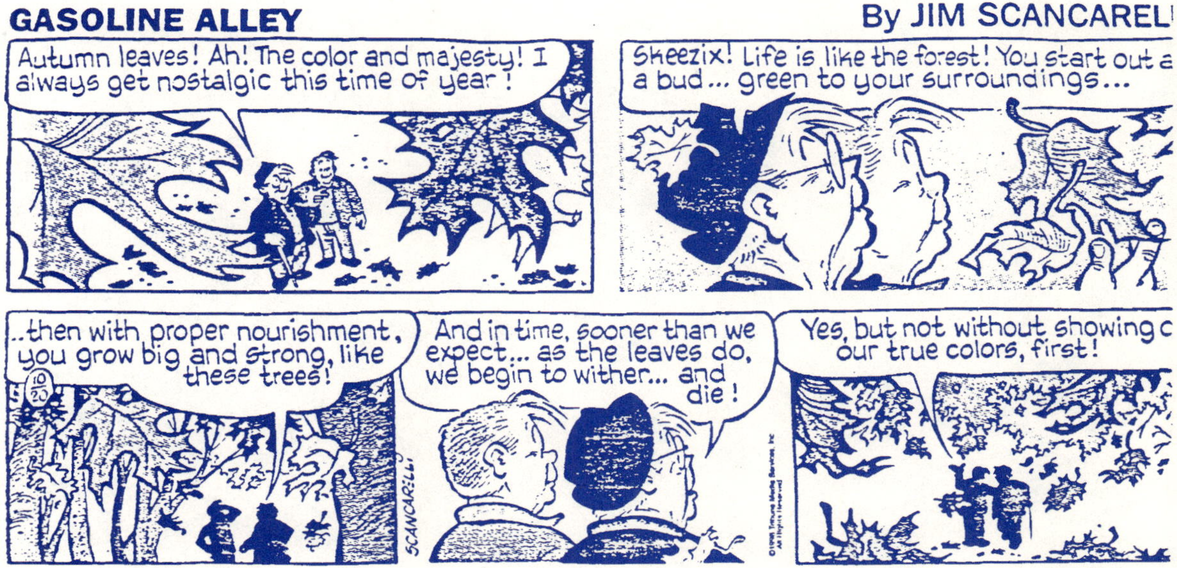
GASOLINE ALLEY
By JIM SCANCAREL
Autumn leaves! Ah! The color and majesty! I always get nostalgic this time of year!
Skeezix! Life is like the forest! You start out a
a bud ... green to your surroundings...
..then with proper nourishment, you grow big and strong, like these trees!
And in time, sooner than we expect... as the leaves do, we begin to wither... and die!
Yes, but not without showing c
our true colors, first!

# *Part 4*
# MEDITATIONS

*You are invited to meditate on these quotations individually, as you chose the ones which best suit you, and to write your thoughts about them.*

*Each person handles pain the way that is best for him or her. There is no right or wrong way. I am sensitive to the needs of others as well as myself.*

*The author extends most profound gratitude to Louise Hay, author of* You Can Do It *(1996-1999) and other books, as well as to Hay House.*

*You are invited to meditate on these quotations individually, as you chose the ones which best suit you, and to write your thoughts about them.*

*My soul cannot be hurt or destroyed; it can only be enriched by whatever my life experiences are.*

*You are invited to meditate on these quotations individually, as you chose the ones which best suit you, and to write your thoughts about them.*

*Laughter is a big part of my life. I freely share my laughter.*

*You are invited to meditate on these quotations individually, as you chose the ones which best suit you, and to write your thoughts about them.*

*Every time I look in the mirror, I give myself a positive message, such as "You are great," "I love you," or "You are wonderful."*

*You are invited to meditate on these quotations individually, as you chose the ones which best suit you, and to write your thoughts about them.*

*The point of power is always in the present moment. I begin—right now—to create new horizons for myself.*

*You are invited to meditate on these quotations individually, as you chose the ones which best suit you, and to write your thoughts about them.*

*I release all unsupportive people from my life. I now surround myself only with friends and relatives whose love, encouragement, and positive energy enhance my life.*

*You are invited to meditate on these quotations individually, as you chose the ones which best suit you, and to write your thoughts about them.*

*I release all addictions to unhealthy people, places and things. I cleanse my body and my mind with healthy doses of self-love and self-esteem.*

*You are invited to meditate on these quotations individually, as you chose the ones which best suit you, and to write your thoughts about them.*

*Several times a day, I breathe deeply and say, "I am aware."*
*Awareness gives me the power to be in charge.*

*You are invited to meditate on these quotations individually, as you chose the ones which best suit you, and to write your thoughts about them.*

*When I experience a problem, I immediately say: "Out of this situation, only good will come. This is easily resolved for the highest good of all concerned."*

*You are invited to meditate on these quotations individually, as you chose the ones which best suit you, and to write your thoughts about them.*

*The most lasting relationship I will ever have is the relationship I have with myself. The one person I am with forever is me.*

*You are invited to meditate on these quotations individually, as you chose the ones which best suit you, and to write your thoughts about them.*

*I put love into those parts of my body that I am not happy with. I love myself inside and out.*

*You are invited to meditate on these quotations individually, as you chose the ones which best suit you, and to write your thoughts about them.*

*I forgive anyone who has ever hurt me. Forgiveness is the key to a joyous existence.*

*You are invited to meditate on these quotations individually, as you chose the ones which best suit you, and to write your thoughts about them.*

*No matter how justified it may seem, I refuse to indulge in damaging emotions and negative thoughts. I think only of what I want to create in my life.*

*You are invited to meditate on these quotations individually, as you chose the ones which best suit you, and to write your thoughts about them.*

*The more I relax, the healthier I am. My body is calm and serene. My exercise program is paying off.*

*You are invited to meditate on these quotations individually, as you chose the ones which best suit you, and to write your thoughts about them.*

*Any time I am presented with a challenge, I know that it is an opportunity to further myself. I quiet my intellect, turn within, and wait for guidance.*

*You are invited to meditate on these quotations individually, as you chose the ones which best suit you, and to write your thoughts about them.*

*I now attract new friends who are exciting, loving, caring, accepting, funny and generous.*

*You are invited to meditate on these quotations individually, as you chose the ones which best suit you, and to write your thoughts about them.*

*I hold my heart tenderly and know that I am doing my best to find my own way through these amazing times that we live in.*

*You are invited to meditate on these quotations individually, as you chose the ones which best suit you, and to write your thoughts about them.*

*The love from my heart flows joyously through my body.*

*You are invited to meditate on these quotations individually, as you chose the ones which best suit you, and to write your thoughts about them.*

*I am the joy of life, expressing and receiving. I am a gift of love.*

*You are invited to meditate on these quotations individually, as you chose the ones which best suit you, and to write your thoughts about them.*

*I make a space in my heart for my inner child to play in. I take time, if only for three minutes, to have a loving conversation with this child and to listen to what it is feeling.*

*You are invited to meditate on these quotations individually, as you chose the ones which best suit you, and to write your thoughts about them.*

*I am independent from the past. I create a powerful, loving, successful life.*

*You are invited to meditate on these quotations individually, as you chose the ones which best suit you, and to write your thoughts about them.*

*Today I observe myself without judgment. I notice what I am thinking at this moment. Is it negative or positive? I simply notice and am aware.*

*You are invited to meditate on these quotations individually, as you chose the ones which best suit you, and to write your thoughts about them.*

*I do random acts of kindness for my fellow human beings without expecting anything in return.*

*You are invited to meditate on these quotations individually, as you chose the ones which best suit you, and to write your thoughts about them.*

*Instead of falling in love, I choose to rise in love. My relationship with my partner grows on many levels each day.*

# *Part 5*

# THE ENDING IS THE BEGINNING

What may seem like an ending may be only the beginning. A peace may come over you like no other you've ever felt; as you listen, reach out your hand, and find your path toward newness of life. From adversity can come advantage. Search for it from your own place. It is yours.

*Our lives are, in a way, question marks. We search for certainty in our world in which there is no certainty, except the certainty of the power of love, and of overcoming.*

I invite you to respond to me with statements of how you dealt with the emotional and spiritual impact of breast cancer. Not the physical, for that is different for each of us, but rather what does this sisterhood consist of.

I would particularly like to know how this book helped you and what made you think, "Yes, that's how I felt." I have given of myself, and hope that you will pass along the gift of compassion.

Renaissance: A New Beginning is the name of my individual and group counseling service. It is available to you wherever you may be, by sending a self-addressed stamped envelope with your letter to me:

Yvonne Buchanan Manley, RN, BS, MA
*Renaissance: A New Beginning*
c/o Hatherleigh Press
5-22 46th Avenue
Long Island City, NY 11101
www.hatherleighpress.com

The following individuals and organizations are remembered here by the author for their personal gifts to her and/or for their gifts to the field of health care.

Dede Cummings, book and cover designer • Fr. Bruce Forbes • Rabbi Allan Schranz • Johnny Hart, creator of *BC* • Syndicates who contributed to breast cancer through the generous use of their material in Healing & Laughter • Louise Hay and Hay House for my healing from her words and for use of *Meditations* • The American Italian Cancer Foundation and The European School of Oncology • The Susan G. Komen Breast Cancer Foundation • Gilda's Club and Gene Wilder • Sisters Network, Inc. • Zeneca-Barr Pharmaceuticals • Charles Slack • Healthcare Chaplaincy • Jamie Bernard of the New York *Daily News* • Katie Couric, NBC Television • Dr. Max Gomez, WNYW-TV • Fran Schneidau, CBS Newsradio • Danielle Steele • Barbara Delinsky • Robin and Rosamunde Pilcher • Sir Paul McCartney • Walter and Kathy Cronkite • MPH Entertainment • Annenberg School of Communication • Department of Culture and Communication, New York University, and Dr. Neil Postman • School of Medicine, Washington University, Saint Louis • V. Craig Jordan, Ph.D., tamoxifen researcher • Weill Medical College of Cornell University and The Center for Women's Health • Zeev Neuwirth, M.D. • John Ravitz, New York State Assemblyman • Dr. Alexandra Solomon • Contiuum Health Partners • New York Women's Foundation • Robert Butler, M.D. • Ann Taylor, Inc. • Inez Tejada, Oncologic Nurse Clinician • William G. Cahan, M.D., chief of Chest Surgery, Emeritus, Memorial Sloan-Kettering Medical Center • Harvard Women's Health Watch • Oxford Health Plans and its founder, Steven Wiggins, M.B.A. • Blue Cross Senior HMO